Unlock Your Inner Glow

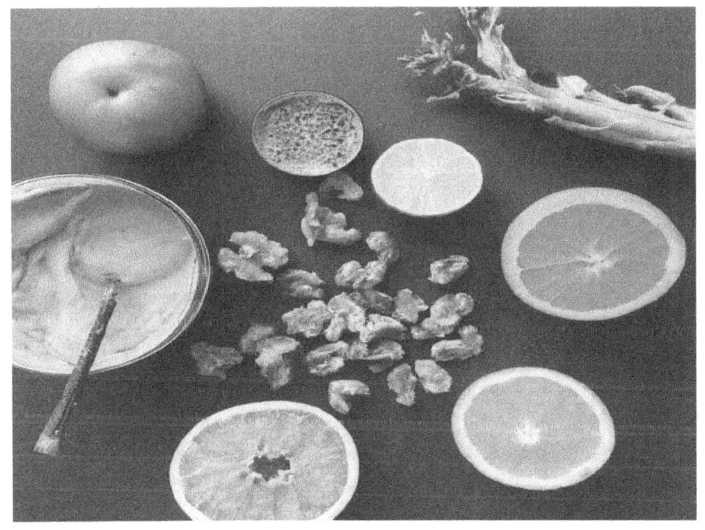

A Detox Cookbook with Delicious Recipes

Tessa Bee

Copyright © [Tesss Bee] [2024]. All rights reserved. No part of this publication may be reproduced, distributed, or transmitted in any form or by any means, including photocopying, recording, or other electronic or mechanical methods, without the prior written permission of the publisher, except in the case of brief quotations embodied in critical reviews and certain other noncommercial uses permitted by copyright law.

Table Of Contents

Introduction

Have you ever craved a radiant complexion that matches the vibrancy you feel inside? In "Unlock Your Inner Glow: A Detox Cookbook with Delicious Recipes," we'll embark on a journey to unveil your natural beauty through the power of detox. This isn't about deprivation or fad diets; it's about nourishing your body with plant-based goodness that fuels a healthy glow from the inside out.

This detox cookbook is your guide to unlocking a brighter, more revitalized you. We'll delve into the connection between what you eat and how you shine. Then, we'll dive into a treasure trove of mouthwatering recipes designed to cleanse your system and tantalize your taste buds. From cleansing broths to vibrant salad bowls and guilt-free treats, "Unlock Your Inner Glow" is packed with delicious recipes that make healthy eating effortless and enjoyable.

Are you ready to shed the dullness and embrace a luminous you? Let's get started!

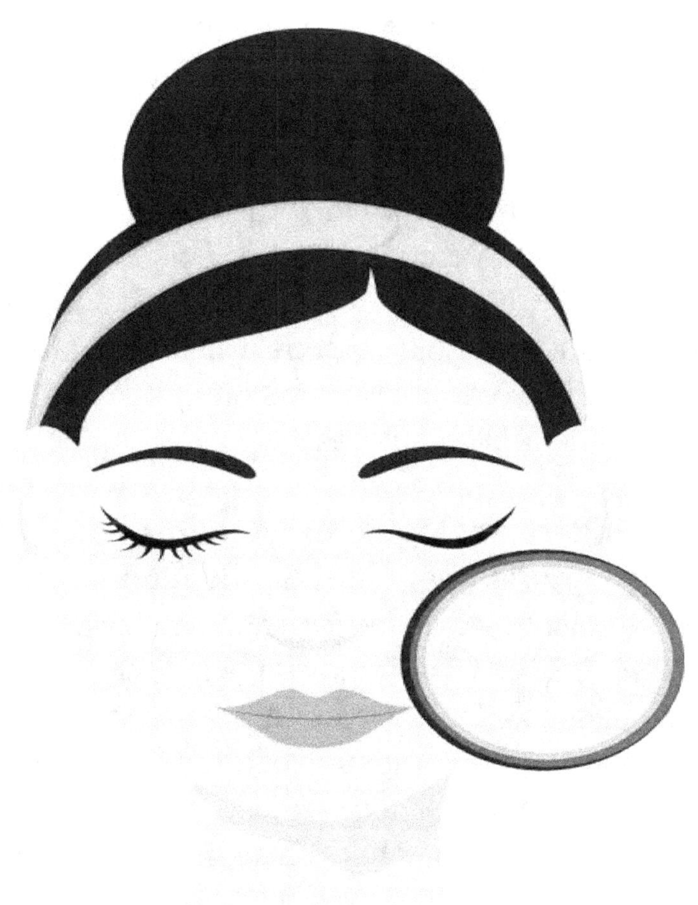

Chapter 1: Unveiling Your Inner Light - The Power of Detox for a Radiant You

Have you ever looked in the mirror and desired a complexion that reflected the lively energy you feel inside? We all have an inner light - a spark of life, pleasure, and well-being that can make us shine. However, daily worries, poor habits, and the accumulation of poisons in our bodies may obscure this glow. This is where detox comes into play, not as a limiting fad diet, but as a powerful tool for restoring our natural beauty and feeling our best.

Understanding detox: A journey of nourishment, not deprivation

Detoxification, or detox for short, is the body's natural process of removing waste products and poisons. Our bodies are very complex machines, with organs such as the liver, kidneys, and intestines working constantly to filter out harmful chemicals. However, the contemporary world throws a lot at us, including processed meals, environmental contaminants, and even stress, which may overwhelm our system and impair its capacity to operate properly. Toxin buildup may occur, resulting in a variety of symptoms, including weariness, poor digestion, acne outbreaks, and a dull complexion.

The Glow Connection: How What You Eat Influences How You Shine.

So, how does what we consume affect all of this? Our food has a significant influence on our general health, including the condition of our skin, our biggest organ. Processed meals, processed carbohydrates, and unhealthy fats may cause inflammation in the body, which can lead to skin issues and a dull complexion. Furthermore, these diets often lack the vital minerals our bodies need to flourish.

On the other hand, eating entire, plant-based meals may improve both our inside and external appearance. Fruits and vegetables are high in vitamins, minerals, antioxidants, and fiber, which all assist our bodies cleanse naturally and perform optimally. Think of vivid fruits and vegetables like leafy greens, berries, citrus fruits, and bell peppers as nature's internal cleaners, washing out impurities and restocking our bodies with nutrition.

Benefits Beyond the Skin: A Comprehensive Approach to Detoxing

While a glowing complexion is a lovely side effect of a detox regimen, the advantages go well beyond the skin. A plant-based detox may cause a variety of good changes:

- Improved Energy Levels: By avoiding processed meals and refined sugars, we can maintain consistent energy levels and prevent weariness.
- Fiber-rich plant-based diets boost gut health, resulting in improved nutrient absorption and digestion.
- Boosted Immunity: Fruits and vegetables include antioxidants and vitamins that help improve the immune system and combat free radicals.
- Mental Clarity: Feeling lethargic might lead to hazy thinking. A detox may assist to boost cognitive function and mental clarity.

Starting Your Detox Journey: Small Steps for Big Results.

To be clear, detox does not have to be a severe transformation that makes you feel starved and unhappy. In reality, making tiny, manageable adjustments that become second nature yields long-term effects. Here are a few recommendations to help you start your detox journey:

- Hydration is essential: Water is a natural detoxifier that flushes away toxins and keeps your body working properly. Drink lots of water throughout the day, and add slices of lemon, cucumber, or ginger for added taste.
- Swap Processed for Fresh: Begin by gradually replacing processed meals with whole, unprocessed alternatives. Think about fresh fruits and veggies, whole grains, legumes, and nuts and seeds.
- Embrace the Power of Plants: Try to integrate more plant-based foods into your diet. Experiment with vegetarian and vegan dishes to explore the delightful world of plant-based nutrition.

- Don't Forget the Fun: Detox does not imply dull meals! This cookbook has a variety of tasty and nutritious dishes. Experimenting with fresh herbs, spices, and taste combinations may make healthy eating enjoyable.

Remember that detox is a journey, not a destination. Be patient with yourself, appreciate your accomplishments, and enjoy the process of providing your body with colorful, tasty food. As you begin on this detox journey, you will not only cleanse your system but also discover your inner glow - a radiance that will leave you feeling confident, invigorated, and vibrantly yourself.

Chapter 2: Plant Power for Your Shine

Have you ever noticed how a stroll through a lush green forest or a bustling flower market awakens your senses? It's not only a coincidence. Plants are nature's powerhouses, packed with life-giving nutrients and antioxidants that contribute to a healthy, radiant you. In this chapter, we'll look at how plant-based diets may help you shine from inside.

Colorful Chemistry of Plants

Plants come alive with a wide variety of hues. The rich reds, oranges, and yellows are powered by carotenoids, potent antioxidants that shield your skin from free radical damage, which is a significant cause of wrinkles and dullness. Carrots, sweet potatoes, red peppers, and luscious mangoes are brimming with these sunshine-colored pigments, ready to brighten your skin.

Do not underestimate the power of green! Chlorophyll, the pigment that gives plants their green tint, is a detoxifying powerhouse. It aids your body's elimination of toxins and waste items, making you feel lighter and fostering a cleaner, more even skin tone. Leafy greens such as kale, spinach, and Swiss chard are high in chlorophyll, while green vegetables such as broccoli and asparagus also contribute significantly.

The vivid blues and purples observed in blueberries, eggplant, and plums are due to anthocyanins, another kind of antioxidant with anti-inflammatory activity. Inflammation may damage your skin, causing redness and discomfort. Incorporating these stunning purple beauties into your diet can help to keep your skin calm and soothed, providing a healthy, balanced shine.

Natural Glow-Getters
Now that we've looked at the vibrant chemistry of plants, let's go further into several crucial elements that will be your constant companions on your inner glow journey:

- Fruits & Berries: Nature's confection contains vitamins, minerals, and antioxidants. Berries, such as strawberries, blueberries, and raspberries, are strong in vitamin C, which is essential for collagen formation, the foundation of healthy, firm skin. Citrus fruits, such as oranges and grapefruits, are high in vitamin C and provide a pleasant source of water.

- Cruciferous Vegetables: Broccoli, cauliflower, and Brussels sprouts may not be the most aesthetically pleasing vegetables, but they carry a big nutritional punch. They contain sulforaphane, a chemical that aids in detoxification and may even provide some UV protection.

- Healthy Fats: Contrary to common thinking, healthy fats are necessary for a glowing complexion. Avocados, almonds, and seeds contain omega-3 and omega-6 fatty acids, which feed skin cells and contribute to a healthy moisture barrier. This results in a smoother, more supple look.

- Whole Grains: Brown rice, quinoa, and whole-wheat bread are not only wonderful for your energy, but they also add to a healthy glow. Whole grains include complex carbs, which give continuous energy throughout the day, avoiding the afternoon slump that may leave you feeling tired and dull.

- Herbs & Spices: Do not underestimate the potency of these taste bombs! Herbs like turmeric and rosemary are high in antioxidants, whilst spices like ginger and cayenne pepper may assist boost circulation, providing critical nutrients to your skin cells for a refreshing flush.

Build Your Plant-Powered Plate.
Now that you've learned about the benefits of plant-based foods, let's use that knowledge to create great meals. Here are some suggestions for creating vivid, glow-boosting plates:

- Color Coordination: Aim to have a rainbow of colors on your plate. This not only assures visual beauty, but also that you are consuming a range of important nutrients.

- Consider "Leafy Greens First": Begin by heaping half your plate with leafy greens like spinach or kale. This puts you on the right track for a nutrient-dense dinner while leaving space for additional delectable items.

- Fiber is Your Friend: Eat lots of fiber-rich foods, such as whole grains, fruits, and vegetables. Fiber keeps you feeling fuller for longer and improves digestion, resulting in a bright, healthy complexion.

- Go for Variety: Don't get locked in a rut! Explore various fruits, veggies, and whole grains to keep your meals interesting and provide a diverse range of nutrients.

Embracing plant power not only nourishes your body, but also invests in your inner radiance. The next chapter will delve into a delightful world of detoxification dishes meant to purify your system and shine your beauty from inside. So prepare to unleash the vivid, brilliant you!

Chapter 3: Detox Delights: Broths, Soups, and Smoothies

Broths, soups, and smoothies serve as the basis for a moderate detox. These nutritious liquids are readily digested, enabling your body to devote its energies to detoxification and renewal. They're high in vitamins, minerals, and antioxidants, which help with detoxification while leaving you feeling invigorated and satiated.

In this chapter, we will look at a range of detox pleasures that are both tasty and detoxifying.

Broths are the foundation of your detox journey.

Broths are the most basic kind of liquid sustenance, and they provide an excellent foundation for many detox dishes. Broths, which are made by cooking vegetables, herbs, and spices in water, are high in taste and provide critical nutrients. They are very hydrating, assisting in the evacuation of impurities, and their warmth may be comfortable and relaxing.

Here are some basic broths to get you started:

- Classic Vegetable Broth: This flexible broth may be enjoyed on its own or used as a foundation for soups and stew. Simply add chopped veggies such as carrots, onions, celery, and garlic with your preferred herbs (bay leaves, thyme, parsley) and cook in water for at least an hour.

- Luminous Lemon Ginger soup: Give your detox a zesty boost with this bright soup. Ginger promotes digestion and contains anti-inflammatory qualities, whilst lemon provides brightness and improves vitamin C levels.

- Superfood Green Broth: Leafy greens are detoxifying agents. Add kale, spinach, or Swiss chard to your soup for an added boost of vitamins and minerals.

Soups: Comforting Cleansers

Soups take your broth to the next level, providing a more substantial and enjoyable detox meal. Simply combine cooked veggies and your broth base until smooth for a creamy texture, or add chopped vegetables, legumes, and healthy grains for a heartier choice. Here are some inspirational soup ideas:

- Minestrone Detox Soup: This traditional Italian soup gets a detox makeover. Fill it up with chopped veggies such as zucchini, carrots, and bell peppers. For protein, include white beans or lentils.

- Spicy Detox Lentil Soup: This bright soup is full of flavor and detoxifying properties. Lentils are high in plant-based protein and fiber, while spices such as cumin, turmeric, and cayenne help with digestion and metabolism.

- Creamy Roasted Cauliflower Soup: Roasting cauliflower highlights its inherent sweetness. Puree it with your favorite broth and a dash of plant-based milk to make a silky smooth, filling soup.

Sprinkle with nutritional yeast for a cheesy taste boost.

Smoothies: On the Go Detox Power

Smoothies are an easy and portable method to get a high dosage of detoxifying substances into your day. They are ideal for hectic mornings or a fast lunchtime pick-me-up.

Here are some smoothie mixes that could boost your inner glow:

- Green Glow Smoothie: This vivid smoothie is loaded with vitamins and minerals. For a refreshing and invigorating combination, combine spinach or kale, banana, pineapple, and a splash of coconut water.

- Berry Detox Delight: Berries are antioxidant-rich and effective cleansers. Blend frozen berries, a scoop of plant-based protein powder, and unsweetened almond milk to make a delightful and filling smoothie.

- Tropical Detox Dream: This smoothie adds a touch of paradise to your detox regimen. For a tropical flavor, combine mango, pineapple, and papaya with lime juice and coconut water.

Tips to Make the Perfect Detox Broth, Soup, and Smoothie

- Fresh is Best: When feasible, use fresh, organic veggies and fruits in detox meals. This guarantees that you get the greatest quantity of nutrients.

- Spice It Up: Not only can spices offer taste, but they also have cleansing effects. To increase the flavor of your broths, soups, and smoothies, try ginger, turmeric, cayenne pepper, cumin and cinnamon.

- Healthy Fats are Your Friend: Including a healthy fat source in your smoothies improves nutrient absorption and keeps you feeling fuller for longer. Add a spoonful of chia seeds, flaxseeds, or avocado for a creamy texture and extra health benefits.

- Proper hydration is essential for detoxification. Aim to drink lots of water throughout the day, in addition to broths, soups, and smoothies.

- Listen to Your Body: While this chapter includes a range of recipes, feel free to experiment and tailor them to your tastes and dietary requirements.

With these tasty and purifying broths, soups, and smoothies, you may go on a journey to rediscover your inner radiance. Remember that consistency is crucial. By including these nutritious drinks into your daily routine, you'll be well on your way to a healthier, more radiant you!

Chapter 4: Salad Bowls and Glowing Meals.

Salad bowls may conjure up visions of limp lettuce and a sprinkle of cherry tomatoes, but in this chapter, we'll turn them into colorful, flavor-packed masterpieces that fuel your body and boost your inner glow. These aren't your typical side dishes; they're full, fulfilling dinners packed with fresh ingredients and vibrant textures.

The Power of Greens:
Let's start with the basics: the greens themselves! Don't settle with iceberg lettuce. Explore the universe of leafy greens, including kale, spinach, arugula, and a combination of the three. Kale has a lot of vitamins A, C, and K, while spinach is high in iron and folate. Arugula provides a peppery taste while also being a high source of vitamin C.

Build Your Bowl:
Now comes the fun part: constructing your bowl! Consider it a blank canvas, ready for your

creative touch. Here are some crucial factors to consider:

- Veggies in all their glory: welcome a burst of color! Bell peppers, carrots, cherry tomatoes, cucumbers, and radishes - their brilliant colors are not only visually appealing, but each vegetable has a distinct combination of nutrients. Roasted veggies offer a hint of caramelized sweetness, and raw vegetables provide a crisp crunch.

- Protein Powerhouses: Add protein to your salad to make it a balanced meal. Grilled chicken breast, sliced tofu, chickpeas, tempeh, and even a dab of Greek yogurt are all excellent choices.

- Whole grains, such as quinoa, brown rice, or farro, give long-lasting energy and keep you content.

- good Fats: Don't avoid good fats! Add sliced avocado, a drizzle of olive oil, or a sprinkling of nuts and seeds. Healthy fats promote nutrition absorption and a sense of fullness.

- Flavorful Toppings: Dress up your salad with delectable toppings. Crumbled feta cheese, dried cranberries, chopped fresh herbs, or a sprinkling of nutritional yeast add variety to your dish.

Dressing up Your Masterpiece:

The dressing is the finishing touch that brings everything together. Avoid store-bought dressings that are high in sugar and bad fats. Instead, make a simple vinaigrette with olive oil, balsamic vinegar, lemon juice, honey, and your favorite herbs. For a creamy alternative, combine avocado with fresh herbs and a squeeze of lemon for a tangy twist.

Sample glowing bowls:

Here are some inspirational salad bowl combos to spark your creativity:

- Mediterranean Glow Bowl: Begin with a bed of baby spinach. Add the sliced cucumber, diced red onion, crumbled feta cheese, kalamata olives, and sun-dried tomatoes. Garnish with grilled chicken breast pieces and a lemon-tahini dressing.

- Spicy Thai Crunch Bowl: Fill a bowl with shredded romaine lettuce, julienned carrots, red bell pepper, and bean sprouts. Add the crumbled tofu, which has been marinated and pan-fried with soy sauce and chili flakes. Finish with chopped peanuts, sweet chili sauce, and lime.

- Summer Berry Quinoa Bowl: Mix together fluffy quinoa, mixed greens, fresh berries like blueberries and raspberries, crumbled goat cheese, and toasted almonds. Drizzle with a mild honey-lemon vinaigrette.

- Rainbow Veggie Power Bowl: Roast a variety of veggies, including sweet potatoes, broccoli florets, and red onions. Combine them with massaged kale, chickpeas, hemp seeds, and a vivid lemon-ginger dressing.

Beyond greens:

Salad dishes aren't only for greens! Consider using spiralized zucchini noodles, cauliflower rice, or even roasted sweet potato cubes as a basis. Get creative and have fun experimenting!

Remember, don't be scared to improvise! Customize these recipes depending on your tastes and what is in season.

By embracing nature's abundance and allowing your creativity to flow, you can convert ordinary salad bowls into delectable, nutrient-dense meals that will give you a bright glow both inside and out.

Chapter 5: Sweet Detox Treats: Indulge without Guilt.

Let's face it: cravings are a normal part of any detox program. However, opting for sugary goodies might derail your efforts and make you feel lethargic. Fear not, detox warriors! This chapter is a refuge for sweet delicacies that satiate your needs while remaining true to your inner glow objective.

These meals are made with healthy components that will feed your body. We will replace processed sugars with natural sweeteners such as dates, maple syrup, and ripe fruits. Don't worry, they won't make you feel starved. These delights are full of taste and deliver a pleasant amount of sweetness.

Chocolate bliss balls:
These bite-sized powerhouses are ideal for a rapid energy boost. They're high in healthy fats, fiber, and antioxidants, which will keep you energetic and suppress your sweet desire.

Ingredients:

- 1 cup rolled oats.
- 1/2 cup chopped almonds.
- 1/2 cup pitted dates.
- 1/4 cup unsweetened cocoa powder.
- 1/4 cup nut butter (almond or peanut).
- 2 tablespoons chia seeds.
- 1/4 cup of unsweetened almond milk.

Instructions:
- In a food processor, blend the oats, almonds, and dates until finely ground.
- Combine cocoa powder, nut butter, and chia seeds. Pulse to mix.
- Drizzle in almond milk one tablespoon at a time, pounding in between additions, until a sticky dough forms.
- Roll the dough into 1-inch balls. Arrange on a baking sheet coated with parchment paper.
- Refrigerate for a minimum of 30 minutes before serving.

Spiced apple crisp with oatmeal crumble:

This traditional comfort dish gets a detox makeover. The crunchy oat crumble and juicy, cinnamon-scented apples make an excellent combo, and the best part? There's no guilt involved!

Ingredients:

For the apples:
- 4 big apples, peeled, cored, and thinly sliced.
- 1/4 cup fresh squeezed orange juice.
- 1/4 cup water.
- 1/4 teaspoon of ground cinnamon.
- 1/8 teaspoon of ground nutmeg.
- 2 tablespoons maple syrup.
- For the oatmeal crumble:
- 1/2 cup rolled oats.
- 1/4 cup chopped walnuts.
- 2 tablespoons ground flaxseed.
- 1 tablespoon of heated coconut oil.
- One tablespoon maple syrup.
- 1/4 teaspoon of ground cinnamon.
- A pinch of sea salt.

Instructions:

- Preheat the oven to 375° Fahrenheit (190° Celsius). Lightly butter an 8x8-inch baking dish.

For the apples: In a large saucepan, mix the apples, orange juice, water, cinnamon, nutmeg, and maple syrup. Bring to a boil, then cover and cook for 10-12 minutes, or until the apples have softened somewhat.

Oat Crumble: In a medium mixing bowl, add oats, walnuts, flaxseed, coconut oil, maple syrup, cinnamon, and salt. Mix until crumbly.
- Pour the apple mixture into the prepared baking dish.
- Distribute the oat crumble evenly over the apples.
- Bake for 20-25 minutes, or until the crumble becomes golden brown and the apples bubble.
- Allow to cool slightly before serving.

Creamy Coconut-Mango Popsicles:

On a hot day, these delicious popsicles are the ideal way to cool off while also satisfying your sweet taste. They're high in vitamin C and good fats, making them a delightful and nutritious treat.

Ingredients:
- One ripe mango, peeled and cut
- 1 cup unsweetened coconut milk.
- 1/4 cup honey.
- 1/2 teaspoon of vanilla essence.

Instructions:
- In a blender, mix the mango, coconut milk, honey, and vanilla essence. Blend until smooth.
- Pour the mixture into the popsicle molds. Freeze for at least 4 to 6 hours, or until solid.

Pro tip: Be creative with your popsicle flavors! Mango may be substituted with other fruits such as strawberries, pineapple, or peaches.

Bonus Recipe: Spicy Roasted Chickpea Clusters.

Craving something salty and crunchy? Roasted chickpea clusters are a healthier alternative to chips. They're high in protein and fiber, and the spicy flavor gives a nice bite.

Ingredients:
- 1 can (15 oz) of chickpeas, drained and rinsed
- 1 tablespoon of olive oil.
- 1/2 teaspoon of chili powder.
- 1/4 teaspoon of smoked paprika.
- 1/4 teaspoon ground cumin.
- 1/8 teaspoon of cayenne pepper (optional)
- A pinch of sea salt.

Instructions:

- Preheat the oven to 400° F (200° C). Line a baking sheet with parchment paper.
- Dry the chickpeas with a clean kitchen towel. This ensures that they crisp up properly.
- In a medium mixing bowl, combine the chickpeas, olive oil, chili powder, paprika, cumin, cayenne pepper (if using), and salt.
- Spread the chickpeas evenly on the prepared baking sheet, arranging them in a single layer. Do not overcrowd the pan; this will prevent them from crisping.

- Bake for 25–30 minutes, tossing regularly, until golden brown and crispy.
- Allow to cool somewhat before consuming.

Here are a few ideas to get your creative juices going. Remember, there are many alternatives for making nutritious and tasty detox treats. Don't be scared to experiment with various ingredients and tastes! Here are some extra strategies for keeping your sweet craving under control throughout your detox:

- Eat lots of fruits: Nature's candy has natural sweetness and fiber, which helps you feel full and reduces cravings.
- Spice things up: Adding cinnamon, nutmeg, and ginger to your meals may provide a hint of sweetness without the sugar rush.
- Drink herbal tea: Unsweetened herbal teas such as peppermint or chamomile might assist with cravings and offer a soothing routine.

- Plan ahead: Having nutritious food on hand can help you avoid reaching for harmful alternatives when cravings arise.

Remember that cleansing is about fueling your body and feeling great. By including these sweet delights into your detox plan, you may fulfill your cravings while staying on track with your objectives. Go forth and detox with a grin (and a tasty goodie in hand)!

Conclusion

You've reached the end of your detox journey with "Unlock Your Inner Glow." By incorporating these delicious, plant-based recipes into your routine, you've not only cleansed your body but nurtured your inner radiance.

Remember, detoxing is a continuous practice, not a one-time event. Keep these principles close to your heart: nourish your body with wholesome foods, prioritize self-care, and celebrate your journey towards a healthier, more vibrant you.

This book is just the beginning. Keep exploring the world of plant-based cuisine, experiment with flavors, and continue to discover the power of food to transform your well-being. As you go forth, let your inner glow continue to shine brightly!